THE GLUCOSE CODE

A Life-Changing Path to Blood Sugar Harmony. Crafting a Life of Wellness, Nourishing Your Body and Energizing Your Life in the Glucose Revolution

By

Mark R. Dickson

Disclaimer

Copyright © by Mark R. Dickson 2024.
All rights reserved.

Table Of Contents

Disclaimer

Introduction

Chapter 1: What Exactly is Glucose?

Steps Taken by Your Body to Metabolize Glucose

When and How to Test Your Glucose

Ranges You Should Anticipate to Find Glucose in Your Body

Expected Outcomes if Your Glucose Levels Are Not Appropriately Managed

Chapter 2: Controlling Your Blood Sugar Levels

How to Determine Your Blood Sugar Level

Treatment Options for Low Blood Sugar

Therapy Options for High Blood Sugar

Things You can do to Help keep your Blood Sugar Levels in Control

Chapter 3: How to Reduce the Peaks and Valleys in Your Blood Sugar Levels Naturally

Why Reducing Blood Sugar Spikes?

Chapter 4: The Power of Nutrition

Comprehensive Guide to Blood-Sugar-Friendly Foods.

Impact of Carbohydrates, Fats, and Proteins on Blood Sugar.

Sample Meal Plans and Recipes

Chapter 5: Exercise and Blood Sugar Control

How Physical Activity Can Positively Influence Blood Sugar Levels

Recommended Exercise For Individuals With Different Fitness Levels

Benefits of Incorporating Both Aerobic and Resistance Training

Chapter 6: Lifestyle Changes for Blood Sugar Balance

Importance of Sleep, Hydration, and other Lifestyle Factors.

Practical Tips for Incorporating Healthy Habits Into Daily Life

Chapter 7: Mindful Living and Stress Reduction

The Connection Between Stress and Blood Sugar Levels

Mindfulness Techniques and Stress Reduction Strategies

Importance of Mental Well-Being in Overall Health.

Conclusion

Introduction

You may not even notice any changes if you keep a tight eye on your glucose levels. However, when they become extremely low or high, they have the ability to disrupt your body's natural functioning.

The word "glucose" comes from the Greek word "glucose." This type of sugar, which comes from the meals you eat, is converted by your body into energy. As it travels via your circulatory system to your cells, it is referred to as blood glucose or blood sugar.

Insulin is a hormone that carries glucose from the bloodstream into the body's cells, where it can be used for energy or stored. Diabetes patients have much higher blood glucose levels than the general population. They either do not have enough insulin to pass through their system, or their cells do not respond to insulin as well as they should.

Glucose is a molecule with the chemical formula $C_6H_{12}O_6$ and six carbon atoms. It is an energy source that can be found everywhere.

It is found in every organism on the planet and is required for aerobic and anaerobic cellular respiration to work effectively. The isometric forms of glucose that enter the body include galactose and fructose (monosaccharides), lactose and sucrose (disaccharides), or starch. Starch (polysaccharides) can also enter the body as glucose. When we go without food for an extended period of time, our bodies release glucose that had previously been stored as glycogen, a glucose polymer. Gluconeogenesis is a mechanism that allows glucose to be created from byproducts of fatty acid and protein degradation. Given the importance of glucose in maintaining homeostasis, it should come as no surprise that there are numerous sources of glucose.

Glucose is carried throughout the blood and then to the tissues that demand energy as soon as it enters the body. Glucose is digested at that site via a series of metabolic events that result in the creation of ATP and the release of energy. The ATP produced by these processes is subsequently used to power almost every other activity in the body that requires energy. Aerobic activities, which need the presence of oxygen and begin with a glucose molecule, provide the majority of the energy required by eukaryotic cells. The glucose is initially digested by the anaerobic process known as glycolysis, which produces some ATP as well as pyruvate as an end product. When anaerobic conditions exist, pyruvate initiates a reduction process that culminates in lactate formation. Under aerobic conditions, pyruvate can enter the citric acid cycle, resulting in the creation of energy-rich electron carriers that contribute to the production of ATP at the electron transport chain.

Chapter 1: What Exactly is Glucose?

Glucose, often referred to as blood sugar, is a fundamental molecule that serves as a primary source of energy for the human body. It plays a central role in the intricate dance of biochemical processes that sustain life. At its core, glucose is a simple sugar—a carbohydrate composed of six carbon atoms, twelve hydrogen atoms, and six oxygen atoms, chemically represented as $C_6H_{12}O_6$.

This remarkable molecule is not just a passive participant in our metabolic orchestra; it's a vital player that fuels our cells, tissues, and organs. When we consume carbohydrates through food, our digestive system breaks them down into glucose, which is then absorbed into the bloodstream. This surge of glucose triggers the pancreas to release insulin, a hormone that acts like a key, allowing cells to open up and take in glucose for energy.

The body's ability to maintain an optimal blood glucose level is crucial for overall health. Too much or too little glucose in the bloodstream can have profound consequences. In conditions like diabetes, for instance, the regulation of glucose becomes impaired. The body does not manufacture insulin in type 1 diabetes, resulting in elevated blood sugar levels. In type 2 diabetes, the body's cells become resistant to insulin, resulting in a similar outcome.

The importance of glucose extends beyond its role as an energy source. It serves as a critical component in various biological processes, such as the synthesis of DNA, RNA, and proteins. The brain, in particular, heavily relies on a steady supply of glucose for optimal functioning. When blood glucose levels drop, individuals may experience symptoms such as fatigue, irritability, and difficulty concentrating—a phenomenon commonly known as hypoglycemia.

While glucose is undeniably essential for life, maintaining a delicate balance is key. Chronic high levels of blood glucose can contribute to the development of various health issues, including cardiovascular diseases, kidney problems, and nerve damage. On the other hand, consistently low levels can lead to energy deprivation, impairing the body's ability to function optimally.

Glucose is more than just a sugar; it's a vital currency of energy that keeps the intricate machinery of the human body humming along. Understanding its role in our physiology is crucial for promoting overall health and well-being. From the fueling of daily activities to the sustenance of complex biological processes, glucose is an unsung hero in the symphony of life.

Steps Taken by Your Body to Metabolize Glucose

In a perfect world, your body would use glucose several times every day.

When you put food in your mouth, your body immediately begins processing glucose and other carbohydrates. The pancreas then supports the enzymes in starting the process of breaking down the molecules.

According to 2021 research, the pancreas is an important aspect of how your body processes glucose. The pancreas is the organ in charge of producing hormones such as insulin. When you eat, your body tells the pancreas to secrete insulin to keep up with the rising level of sugar in your blood.

The glucose is subsequently used as fuel by muscle, fat, and other cells, or it is stored as fat for later use.

Diabetes is a disorder that occurs when the pancreas is unable to make enough insulin. In this case, you may require assistance from an outside source (insulin injections) to process and control your body's glucose levels.

Diabetes may also be caused by insulin resistance, according to the conclusions of a 2018 review. This syndrome arises when the cells in the body are unable to detect insulin, resulting in an overabundance of sugar in the bloodstream.

When the body does not respond appropriately to insulin, it stops glucose from entering cells and being used as a source of energy. Your cells manufacture ketones as a response, which indicates their synthesis when you fast or diet, as well as at night.

Insulin resistance, according to the American Diabetes Association, can cause insulin levels to diminish over time. Diabetes complications (ADA) can result from this. Fat may also be liberated from cells in your body that store it. Furthermore, the liver continues to create extra ketones, lowering the pH of your blood to an acidic level.

When the body is unable to use glucose as well as it should, a potentially deadly accumulation of ketones and a shift in blood pH can develop, according to the ADA. The medical word for this condition is ketoacidosis. Diabetes can cause this severe consequence, which endangers a person's life and demands immediate medical intervention.

Diabetes and the Ketogenic Diet

The keto diet has gained popularity, although it is a medical diet with certain potential adverse effects. According to a 2019 study, adopting a ketogenic or low-carbohydrate diet may help people lose body weight; however, those with diabetes or using specific medications may increase their risk of getting ketoacidosis.

Everyone is at risk of extra unfavorable consequences, such as higher cholesterol levels, which are connected to cardiovascular disease. It is in your best interest to see your doctor before commencing any type of diet plan to assist limit the chance of consequences.

When and How to Test Your Glucose

The American Diabetes Association advises diabetics to keep a close eye on their blood glucose levels. Individuals with diabetes should check their blood sugar levels at intervals and periods chosen by their specific needs and goals.

Checking the following numbers on a regular basis will help you keep your glucose levels under control:. Both before and after meals. Prior to and following exercise. When engaging in extended or vigorous physical activity. Before going to bed. When starting therapy with new drugs or a new insulin regimen. When establishing a new work schedule. When traveling over several time zones. It is critical to discuss your glucose level targets with your primary care physician because they are affected by your illness as well as other factors such as your age and medical history.

According to the National Institute of Diabetes and Digestive and Kidney Diseases (NIDDK), one of the most popular ways to monitor one's blood glucose levels at home when living with diabetes is to perform a simple blood test. You perform the following when you use a blood glucose meter:

To draw a drop of blood, make a small puncture on the side of your fingertip using a lancet needle. Place a small amount of blood on the testing strip. Place the strip in the meter............ The meter will tell you how much glucose is in your blood at that particular instant. Glucose monitoring in real time
When it comes to controlling your diabetes, you may want to talk to your primary care provider about adopting a continuous glucose monitoring

(CGM) system. The device will automatically monitor your glucose levels around the clock.

The readings are delivered to a monitor via a very small sensor implanted just beneath the skin's surface, usually on the stomach or the arm. A CGM continuously monitors and records your blood glucose levels, and it will sound an alarm if either level becomes dangerously high or low.

Some of the benefits of using the gadget are as follows:
Fewer finger punctures are required, which aids in improved glucose management and, as a result, fewer medical emergencies.

Ranges You Should Anticipate to Find Glucose in Your Body

It is critical to keep your blood glucose levels within the usual range in order for your body to function properly. People who already have diabetes may need considerably more care and attention.

According to a 2021 review, those who do not have diabetes should have a blood glucose level of less than 100 mg/dL on an empty stomach. It should be less than 140 mg/dL two hours after a meal.

As previously stated, glucose target levels for patients with diabetes vary because they are adjusted to the specific circumstances of each individual patient. Your healthcare practitioner will work with you to create treatment objectives.

This points to several possible causes of high blood sugar levels. Some examples of triggers are:

- 1. Sunburn: The discomfort caused by a sunburn causes stress, which can raise blood sugar levels.
- 2. Coffee: Any amount of coffee, especially black coffee, can make you

more susceptible to caffeine's effect on blood glucose levels.

- 3. Skipping breakfast: Skipping breakfast may result in an increase in blood sugar levels after lunch and dinner.
- 4. The time of day: As the day progresses, your body's ability to control how much glucose it utilizes becomes more challenging. The dawn phenomenon refers to the rise in blood sugar that happens early in the morning. It is produced by the hormonal surge that happens at that time.
- 5. Drugs: Certain drugs and nasal sprays can either cause your liver to create more glucose or prevent it from making insulin. This can happen if some drugs cause the liver to malfunction.
- 6. Tension: Excessive worry and pressure have been connected to blood glucose rises.
- This can also happen if you eat less calories than your body requires on a regular basis, or if you exercise for a

longer period of time or with greater intensity than usual.

In some situations, it has been reported to happen in persons who do not have diabetes.
A meal or a glass of juice may be beneficial in boosting blood glucose levels. If your glucose level falls too low (or climbs too high), your doctor may help you devise a plan that involves keeping glucose supplements on hand.

If hypoglycemia is not treated promptly, it can be fatal. If this occurs, you may require immediate medical assistance.

Hyperglycemia
High levels of glucose in the blood are referred to as hyperglycemia. This could happen if your body lacks insulin or is unable to use insulin adequately.

The American Diabetes Association considers a blood glucose level of more than 130 mg/dL before eating to be above the desired range. Furthermore, the ADA recommends aiming for a range of 180 mg/dL one to two hours after eating. You should speak with your doctor about the target ranges that are appropriate for you.

If you suspect hyperglycemia, keep an eye out for the following symptoms:

- High levels of glucose in the urine
- frequent urination, and
- an increased thirst.

Your normal blood glucose range is determined by a variety of things. Consultation with your physician is the greatest approach to ensure that you are working within a healthy range for yourself.

Aside from uncontrolled diabetes, there are other reasons for hyperglycemia. Unpredictability in diabetes care, for example, may be caused by stress and worry in people with diabetes. This can result in greater glucose levels in the blood.

A nutritious diet and regular exercise can also help keep blood sugar levels in the usual range. However, in other circumstances, physical activity may not be the best option, and insulin may be required instead.

Expected Outcomes if Your Glucose Levels Are Not Appropriately Managed

If your glucose levels are not adequately regulated over time, your body will experience unfavorable consequences. If your blood glucose levels are continuously high, you may get the following symptoms:

- Numbness and tingling in the hands and feet Heart disease
- Decreased vision
- Skin infections, and
- Pain in the joints and limbs.

Coma brought on by extreme dehydration

Diabetes can also cause ketoacidosis and hyperglycemic hyperosmolar syndrome, which are both serious consequences. Diabetes is linked to both disorders in some way.

These symptoms can be caused by a syndrome known as hypoglycemia unawareness.
It keeps you from detecting the signs of low blood glucose until it is really low.

If it falls too low, you risk feeling the following:

- A state of being unconscious
- Coma, as well as
- Death will occur at some point.

Chapter 2: Controlling Your Blood Sugar Levels

Your blood sugar target is the range of blood sugar that you want to strive for as much as feasible. It is critical to keep your blood sugar levels as close to normal as possible in order to help prevent or delay long-term, major health problems, including as heart disease, eyesight loss, and kidney disease. Maintaining your stance inside the range you've selected for yourself might also help you feel more energetic and in a better mood. The following is a list of frequently asked diabetes-related blood sugar questions and answers.

How to Determine Your Blood Sugar Level

A blood sugar meter, also known as a glucometer, or a continuous glucose monitor, abbreviated as CGM, can be used to check your blood sugar. A little amount of blood is drawn from the fingertip and placed into a blood sugar meter, which calculates the amount of sugar in the sample. A continuous glucose monitor (CGM) takes blood sugar readings every few minutes using a sensor implanted under the skin. If you use a CGM, you must still test your blood sugar levels with a blood sugar meter on a daily basis to ensure that the values provided by your CGM are accurate.

When to Check Your Blood Sugar level

The frequency with which you check your blood sugar is dictated by the kind of diabetes you have and whether or not you take diabetes medication.

The following are some examples of usual times to check your blood sugar: As soon as you open your eyes, and long before you've had anything to eat or drink. Just before lunch. After digesting a meal for two hours. Before going to bed.

If you have type 1 diabetes, type 2 diabetes, and use insulin, or if you have low blood sugar frequently, your doctor may advise you to check your blood sugar more frequently, such as before and after physical exercise. If you have type 1 or type 2 diabetes and use insulin, or if you frequently have low blood sugar levels.

Goals and Targets of Blood Sugar Level

A blood sugar target is a range within which you attempt to reach the highest achievable blood sugar levels. Typical goals include the following:

A range of 80 to 130 mg/dL is appropriate before eating.
Blood levels of less than 180 mg/dL two hours after the start of a meal.
Your blood sugar goals may fluctuate depending on a number of factors, such as your age, the

severity of any other health conditions you have, and other circumstances. Discuss your health goals with your health care team members to establish which goals are appropriate for you.

Factors that cause low blood sugar

Low blood sugar, also known as hypoglycemia, can be caused by a number of circumstances, including skipping a meal, taking too much insulin or another diabetic medicine, exercising more than usual, drinking alcohol, or not eating enough. A blood glucose level of less than 70 mg/dL is considered low.

Low blood sugar symptoms might vary considerably from person to person. Some of the most prevalent symptoms are as follows:

An hyperactive nervous system causes trembling, perspiration, uneasiness or anxiety, irritability or perplexity, dizziness, and hunger.
It is critical to be aware of your individual symptoms in order to quickly diagnose and treat

low blood sugar. Even if you don't feel sick, you should have your blood sugar checked if you suspect it's too low. A critically low blood sugar level necessitates rapid medical treatment to be treated.

Treatment Options for Low Blood Sugar

Hypoglycemia Ignorance

If you have previously experienced hypoglycemia unawareness, which means that you have low blood sugar without feeling or seeing any symptoms, you may need to check your blood sugar more regularly to identify if it is low and then treat it. Driving with low blood sugar is dangerous, so check your blood sugar before getting behind the wheel.

Carry the supplies you'll need to treat low blood sugar. If you are experiencing symptoms like as shakiness, sweating, intense hunger, or any other symptoms, check your blood sugar. If you suspect you have low blood sugar, even if you don't have any symptoms, check your blood sugar level.

If your blood sugar is less than 70 mg/dL, you should do one of the following right away:

Take four glucose pills in total.
Squeeze four ounces of fruit juice into your mouth. It is advised to drink four ounces of regular soda rather than diet soda.
Consume four individual hard candy pieces.
Check your blood sugar level once more after fifteen minutes.
Repeat any of the above therapies until your blood sugar reaches at least 70 mg/dL, and make sure to take a snack if your next meal is more than an hour away. If you experience low blood sugar problems, consult your doctor to see if your treatment plan has to be changed.

Factors that lead to blood sugar increase

A high blood sugar level, commonly known as hyperglycemia, can be caused by a number of circumstances, including illness, stress, eating more than planned, or forgetting to deliver enough insulin. When left untreated, high blood sugar can lead to serious health problems that last for a long time.

High blood sugar symptoms include the following:

- I'm feeling quite exhausted. quench one's thirst with.
- Having an ambiguous vision.
- Having a greater need to urinate (or pee).

Maintaining a healthy blood sugar level can be difficult when you're unwell. It is conceivable that you will not be able to ingest as much food or liquid as usual, which may affect your blood sugar levels. If you are unwell and your blood sugar is 240 mg/dL or above, you should examine your urine for ketones using an over-the-counter ketone test kit. If your ketones are elevated, you should consult your doctor. An increased amount of ketones may be an early warning indication of diabetic ketoacidosis, a medical emergency that necessitates prompt care.

What are ketones, exactly?
When fat is broken down for energy, a byproduct known as ketones is created. When you don't have enough insulin in your bloodstream, your liver will start breaking down fat to enable blood sugar into your cells. This is known as ketosis.

What precisely is diabetic ketoacidosis?

Even if you don't feel sick, you should have your blood sugar checked if you suspect it's too low.

Ketones can build up in the body and cause diabetic ketoacidosis, commonly known as DKA, if they are produced at an abnormally high rate. Diabetic ketoacidosis (DKA) is a serious illness that can even lead to death. The following are some of the most prevalent DKA symptoms:

- Quickly and deeply inhale and exhale.
- Dryness of the lips and skin The cheeks were flushed.
- Urinating often or experiencing acute thirst for at least a day.
- A strong fruity odor in one's breath.
- Headache.
- Muscle stiffness and pains are common symptoms.
- Nausea and vomiting are symptoms.
- My stomach hurts.

A urine ketones test can help establish whether you have diabetic ketoacidosis (DKA). To calculate your ketone level, follow the instructions included with the test kit and compare the color of the test strip to the color chart included with the kit. If your ketones levels are high, you should see your doctor as soon as possible. Hospitalization is required for DKA treatment.

DKA is most common in patients with type 1 diabetes and can even be the first indicator of the condition in people who haven't been diagnosed. DKA can also occur in patients with type 2 diabetes, however it is considerably less prevalent.

Therapy Options for High Blood Sugar

Make a mental note of the following suggestions:

1. Increase your physical exercise. Exercise on a regular basis can help you maintain healthy blood sugar levels. Important: Do not exercise if your urine contains ketones. This can raise your blood sugar even higher than it is already.

2. Follow the medicine instructions exactly. If your blood sugar levels are frequently high, your doctor may modify the dosage or timing of your prescription.

3. Stick to the diabetes food plan you devised. If you are experiencing difficulty sticking to your diet, you should seek the advice of a medical expert or a nutritionist.

4. Check your blood sugar levels on a frequent basis, as instructed by your healthcare practitioner. If you are sick or concerned about high or low blood sugar levels, you should check them more regularly.

Consult your primary care physician about modifying the amount of insulin you take and the type of insulin you use (such as rapid-acting insulin).

What effect do carbohydrates have on blood sugar levels?

When you eat foods high in carbohydrates, your blood sugar levels rise faster than when you eat foods high in proteins or fats. You can ingest carbohydrates even if you have diabetes. Your age, weight, exercise level, and other factors all contribute to how much you can ingest while keeping your desired blood sugar level. Carbohydrate counting is a vital technique for those who want to keep their blood sugar levels under control. To attain the best results, make sure to discuss your carbohydrate objectives with your health care team.

What precisely is an A1C test?

The A1C test is a simple blood test that evaluates your typical blood sugar levels over the past two to three months. The test is performed in a laboratory or at your doctor's office in addition to, and not in place of, your regular blood sugar testing.

The ABCs of diabetes include A1C testing, which are crucial steps you may take to avoid or delay the development of future health complications:

A: Get a routine A1C test.

B: recommended a goal of keeping your blood pressure below 140/90 mm Hg (or the target recommended by your doctor).

C: Keep an eye on your cholesterol levels.

s: Either quit smoking or don't start.

The A1C target range for the vast majority of adults with diabetes is between 7% and 8%, although your target range may vary depending on your age, other health conditions, medications you're taking, and other variables. Work with your healthcare physician to identify an A1C target that is right for you.

Things You can do to Help keep your Blood Sugar Levels in Control

Eating a fruit and vegetable-rich diet, maintaining a healthy weight, and engaging in regular physical activity are all things that can help. Other helpful hints include:

- Keep a record of your blood sugar levels so you can figure out what is causing them to climb or fall.

- Maintain a consistent eating pattern and avoid skipping meals.
- Select foods with fewer calories, saturated fat, trans fat, sugar, and salt.
- Maintain a journal of everything you eat, drink, and do physically.
- Water should be used instead of juice and soda. Limit your intake of alcoholic beverages.
- If you want something sweet to snack on, choose some fruit.

Watch your portion sizes (for example, utilize the plate method: fill half your plate with non-starchy veggies, a quarter with lean protein, and a quarter with a grain or starchy meal).

Why are glucose levels dangerously high?

If you have diabetes, you are aware that blood sugar spikes are typical and that these spikes should be expected. Day-to-day glucose regulation is exceedingly complex due to the plethora of factors involved, including but not limited to nutrition, exercise, stress, hormones, medications (including insulin), and more. You should expect to encounter both the highs of hyperglycemia and the lows of hypoglycemia at some point in your life. This is an unavoidable circumstance.

But why are blood sugar spikes bad for your health, and what can you do to avoid the onset and frequency of high blood sugars?

The specific reasons for high blood sugar levels are discussed in the following paragraphs.

Risky, as well as what you can do to assist prevent them.

What are the Root Causes of a Blood Sugar Spike?

A blood sugar spike occurs when there is an excess of glucose in the bloodstream but not enough insulin to help the cells absorb it properly. Diabetes patients can develop this condition for a variety of reasons, including, but not limited to:

At mealtime, there is insufficient insulin.
Incorrect carbohydrate counting
Carbohydrates sneaked in as sauces, creams, or liquids
Errors with insulin administration Using contaminated insulin
Caffeine consumption is excessive.
Have you lately changed the insulin you're taking or the dosage?
Sickness
Steroids, in combination to other drugs

Being treated for a sickness or having recently undergone surgery, using a transitional basal for exercise, and then failing to exercise for as long or as strenuously as expected
Stress\sHormones

Pregnancy (may result in both high and low blood sugar levels)

Making an impact on insulin resistance

Blood sugar spikes are caused by the following factors:

Whatever way you and your care team decide to define your diabetes goals, the most essential thing is to maintain your blood sugar levels stable and under control at all times.

Even if this isn't always achievable, it's critical to avoid hyperglycemia to the maximum extent possible.

If you have many frequent, short-term rises in your blood sugar, you may be more prone to diabetes fatigue and depression, anxiety, sleep deprivation, and unstable mood changes.

You may also notice more frequent headaches, weight changes, and difficulty sticking to a schedule when it comes to your fitness program, work, school, or social engagements with other people.

This can also have a severe impact on your connections with family and friends, leading to feelings of loneliness and isolation. Because the HbA1c test is simply an average of the previous three months' blood glucose, it is conceivable to have a "good" score that is simply an average of a lot of highs and a lot of lows. This can give you a false sense of accomplishment, leading you to assume that you have succeeded in managing your diabetes when, in fact, you have not.

If you use a continuous glucose monitor, you can also track the amount of time your blood sugar levels are within a specified range (TiR). Collaborate with your healthcare team to decide what percentage of the time they want your blood sugar to be within a given range, and then set a goal to maintain that percentage while also aiming to improve it over time.

Unexpected items can cause a jump in your blood sugar:

You checked your blood sugar levels frequently after discovering that you had diabetes. As a result, you have a greater grasp of how many things, like diet, activity, stress, and sickness, might affect your blood sugar levels. You should have a decent understanding of the problem at this stage. Then, suddenly, bam! Something causes your blood sugar to swiftly spike. It dips to an incredibly low level when you try to modify it with food, activity, or insulin. You're now on a roller coaster that diabetics don't want to ride.

Do you understand everything you need to know about blood sugar triggers?

The expression "knowledge is power" Keep an eye out for the following unexpected factors that can cause your blood sugar to skyrocket:

- Sunburns are excruciating, and this produces stress, which elevates blood sugar levels.

- More research on artificial sweeteners is needed, but some studies have suggested that using them can boost blood sugar levels. Even when no sugar is added to the coffee.

- Caffeine can make some people's blood sugar levels more sensitive than usual.

- Sleep deprivation—even one night of inadequate sleep might lead your body to use insulin less effectively.

- If you skip breakfast, your blood sugar will rise after lunch and dinner, especially if you don't replace it with another meal. When it comes to blood sugar control, the later it is in the day, the more difficult it might be to maintain good control. The dawn phenomenon refers to the increase in hormone levels that happens in persons early in the morning, regardless of whether they have diabetes or not. Diabetes patients are more likely to encounter blood sugar increases.

- Because there is less water in your body when you are dehydrated, your blood sugar becomes more concentrated. Some nasal sprays include ingredients that are harmful to your health.

- Increase the amount of blood sugar produced by your liver. Diabetes increases the likelihood of gum disease, and gum disease can induce a jump in blood sugar levels.

- Keep an eye out for any additional things that could cause a dip in your blood sugar.

- Exposure to extremely high temperatures, for example, can cause blood vessels to enlarge (widen). This causes an increase in insulin absorption, which may result in a drop in blood sugar. Checking your blood sugar levels before and after a new exercise or eating a new food might help you predict how your body will react.

Chapter 3: How to Reduce the Peaks and Valleys in Your Blood Sugar Levels Naturally

We've been working hard over the last few months to boost our immunity while also attempting to smooth out the curves of COVID-19. Consider that every time you drink a cup of green tea, you are strengthening your immune system. "Blood sugar spikes" is another curve to be aware of and monitor. We will discuss how to naturally level off the curve of blood sugar increases in this session.

Despite having normal blood sugar levels, an increasing proportion of people are developing insulin resistance.

You may believe that high blood sugar is only a concern when your blood sugar test results are higher than 120 or when you are diagnosed with diabetes. Despite the fact that one's blood sugar test results may still appear "normal," insulin health may have been affected.

We develop a habit of eating throughout the day because we live in a culture where there is an abundance of ready-to-eat food. When you eat, your blood sugar rises, your pancreas secretes more insulin more frequently, and your body's cells may progressively acquire "insulin resistance." This occurs each time you eat.

Insulin resistance occurs when your body's cells do not respond well to insulin and are unable to easily absorb enough blood sugar from your blood. This causes your pancreas to produce more insulin.
Even if your blood sugar tests show "normal" results, your pancreas may be working twice, three times, or even five times harder to keep up as insulin resistance grows. While your blood sugar tests indicate "normal" readings, your pancreas may be working twice, three times, or even five times harder.

According to "MedlinePlus," a division of the National Library of Medicine in the United States, "initial insulin resistance causes the body to produce extra insulin in order to compensate for ineffective insulin." Hypoglycemia can result from an excess of insulin in the bloodstream. Insulin resistance, on the other hand, tends to deteriorate over time. As a result, your body's ability to manufacture insulin will eventually decline. Blood sugar levels rise as insulin levels fall."

If you do not keep the blood sugar spikes gradual, flattening, and rare, your insulin sensitivity will be exhausted over time.

Why Reducing Blood Sugar Spikes?

The following are some further arguments in favor of keeping the slope low:
The greater the blood sugar level, the more free radicals are created, and these free radicals cause both oxidative and inflammatory damage.

Because insulin blocks leptin, the satiety hormone that informs the brain when it's time to quit eating, from reaching its receptors in the brain, a higher insulin level makes you feel hungrier. As a result, as we consume more food, we grow more hungry.

A greater insulin level also prevents fat from being broken down into its constituent parts and used as an energy source.

There are five things we can take to create large and practically immediate improvements in blood sugar rises.
It is critical to avoid diets high in sugar, processed carbohydrates, and excessive processing. Simultaneously, including more

whole foods and fiber into the diet is a crucial component of the treatment strategy. What are our alternative options? Fortunately, some natural and holistic approaches can have an immediate and favorable impact on the system.

1. Always match your food with the appropriate beverage.
The beverage you drink with your meal can influence how quickly your blood sugar levels rise after you eat. Which one do you think is the most successful in lowering blood sugar spikes?

a) White flour and water bread
b) A loaf of white bread and a glass of red wine
c) The beverage of choice is unadulterated white bread and red wine. Is Green Tea Really Better Than Water?
In the instance of c), the phytochemical components and antioxidants contained in wine aided the blood sugar surge. What do you suppose would happen if you drank green tea instead of wine?

Scientific studies have shown that the antioxidants included in green tea can help prevent blood sugar increases. A different study discovered that the antioxidants in green tea helped to postpone "gastric emptying," but only to a statistically meaningful degree.

The next issue is, what about caffeine? Caffeine may make you less susceptible to the effects of insulin. This suggests that your cells do not absorb as much sugar from your blood after a meal. Your body will need to create more insulin as a result of this.

Green tea is considered a "blood sugar-friendly" beverage option because it has much less caffeine than coffee. Growing up in Japan, the traditional beverage to accompany meals was either a hot cup of tea or a glass of iced tea. Because it is now available in powder form, it is now possible to make an authentic cup of Sencha, Genmaicha, or even Hojicha in seconds.

On the other side, one of my favorite activities is to brew loose leaf tea, either hot or cold, and enjoy both the process and the flavor.

2. Consume Less Unhealthy "Condiments"
If you are not a committed vegetarian but want to reduce the harmful effects of animal protein on your body while still enjoying it on occasion, you can do so by supplementing it with a superfood.
Adding avocado, almonds, berries, or leafy greens to hamburgers, according to research, can minimize the amount of oxidative damage and free radicals created. Green Tea Powder is yet another "super condiment" that can be useful. Green Tea Powder is a pantry staple that we use frequently. The vast majority of our clients advise them to "just sprinkle here and there."

3. Determine the most convenient time for you to exercise.
Adults with metabolic syndrome may benefit from minimizing postprandial metabolic dysfunction by taking dietary polyphenols with a

meal and then engaging in physical exercise after the meal, according to research. According to the study's findings, the intensity of walking does not need to be high in order to cause a fall in blood sugar. Adults can extend this effect by walking after many meals to improve their overall daily glycemic load. This can be accomplished by increasing the amount of time they spend walking overall.

4. Make Certain You Get a Good Night's Sleep

Both stress and lack of sleep contribute to a rise in blood sugar levels. Sleep deprivation also increases the production of the stress hormone cortisol, which can lead to insulin resistance. Other hormones, such as thyroid-stimulating hormone (TSH) and testosterone, are also affected by insomnia, which can lead to impaired insulin sensitivity and higher blood sugar levels.

5. Relax Your Mind

When under stress, it's human nature to go for comfort foods, which can lead to a vicious cycle of overeating. Meditation activates the parasympathetic nerve system, which decreases stress, cortisol, insulin, and sensations of hunger. The parasympathetic nerve system is sometimes referred to as the "rest and digest system." This is because the parasympathetic nervous system is in charge of decreasing the heart rate, increasing bowel and gland activity, and relaxing the sphincter muscles of the gastrointestinal tract.

We hope you have pleasure learning new methods to use green tea to give your meal more vitality and smooth out the curve of blood sugar rises. If you practice intermittent fasting, Herbal Tea is another excellent beverage to explore.

It has been seven months after the first incidence of COVID-19 was verified in the United States on January 20, 2020. The "new normal," characterized by a sense of great unpredictability, has begun to permeate both our thinking and the way we live our lives. Even if returning to what is considered "normal" can be reassuring, there are some "normals" to which we can refuse to return. Maintain your safety and health, and keep pushing forward!

Chapter 4: The Power of Nutrition

Comprehensive Guide to Blood-Sugar-Friendly Foods.

Let's talk about the powerhouse that is nutrition and how it holds the key to unlocking the magic of balanced blood sugar. Forget the confusing jargon and let's break it down like we're chatting over a cup of coffee.

Picture your body as a finely tuned machine, and nutrition is the fuel that keeps it running smoothly. When it comes to blood sugar, the right foods can be your best allies. We're not talking about a strict diet that feels like punishment. Nope, this is about embracing a lifestyle that not only tastes good but also helps keep your blood sugar in check.

First things first, let's get cozy with the term "glycemic index" (GI). It's like the Netflix rating for foods but for your blood sugar. Foods with a high GI are like blockbuster movies—they cause a rapid spike in blood sugar, leaving you crashing later. On the other hand, low-GI foods are like hidden gems, releasing energy more steadily. Think whole grains, sweet potatoes, and legumes – these are the superheroes of the nutrition world.

Now, don't go banishing carbs from your life just yet. Carbs can be your friends, but it's all about choosing the right ones. Opt for complex carbohydrates found in whole grains, fruits, and veggies. They're the reliable buddies that keep your blood sugar on an even keel.

Fiber is another unsung hero. It's like the janitor of your digestive system, sweeping away excess sugar and keeping things tidy. Load up on fiber-rich foods like oats, beans, and veggies. Your gut will thank you, and so will your blood sugar levels.

Let's talk about fats – the good, the bad, and the ugly. Ditch the trans fats; they're the villains wreaking havoc on your health. Instead, embrace the good fats found in avocados, nuts, and olive oil. They're like superheroes protecting your cells and supporting overall well-being.

Proteins are the building blocks of life, and they play a crucial role in blood sugar control. Include lean proteins like poultry, fish, tofu, and legumes in your diet. They not only keep you feeling full and satisfied but also prevent those blood sugar rollercoaster rides.

But hey, life is about balance, right? Treat yourself occasionally. Dark chocolate, anyone? It's not just a guilty pleasure; it contains antioxidants and may even have a positive impact on insulin sensitivity. It's the small indulgences that make the journey enjoyable.

Now, let's navigate the supermarket aisles together. Load up on colorful veggies; they're like a nutrient-packed rainbow for your plate. Explore the world of whole grains – quinoa, brown rice, and whole wheat pasta – they're the reliable sidekicks that keep you energized.

And don't forget the hydration game. Water is the unsung hero in the blood sugar saga. It keeps everything flowing smoothly, helping your body process glucose efficiently. Make friends with herbal teas and infused water for added flavor without the sugar overload.

So, there you have it – a nutrition pep talk that's as real as it gets. Balancing blood sugar isn't about deprivation; it's about making informed, delicious choices. Embrace the power of nutrition, savor the journey, and let your plate be a canvas for a healthier, happier you.

Impact of Carbohydrates, Fats, and Proteins on Blood Sugar.

Ever wondered about the secret dance your food does inside your body? It's like a mini-orchestra, with carbohydrates, fats, and proteins taking center stage. Now, let's dive into the backstage drama of how these players impact the star of the show—your blood sugar.

Carbohydrates:
Think of carbohydrates as the rockstars of the food world. They come in various forms—sugars, starches, and fibers—and have a direct influence on your blood sugar levels. Picture this: you indulge in a sugary doughnut. The carbohydrates from the doughnut quickly break down into sugar (glucose) during digestion, hitting your bloodstream like a burst of confetti. Cue the sudden spike in blood sugar! But wait, there's more to this story. Whole grains, fruits, and veggies are the good guys, releasing their

glucose more gradually, preventing the wild rollercoaster ride of a sugar rush.

Fats:

Ah, the misunderstood rebels of the culinary realm. Fats may not directly impact blood sugar, but they sure play a backstage role in the blood sugar drama. When you consume fat with carbs, it slows down the carb digestion process, creating a smooth, controlled release of glucose into the bloodstream. It's like fats are the cool moderators, making sure the party doesn't get too out of hand. But, and here's the twist, too much of the wrong kind of fats can lead to insulin resistance, where the body struggles to manage blood sugar effectively. So, fats are like backstage managers—essential for the overall performance but need careful supervision.

Proteins:

Meet the builders and repairers of the food world. Proteins are like stagehands working tirelessly behind the scenes, ensuring everything runs smoothly. Unlike carbs, proteins have a minimal impact on blood sugar levels. When you consume protein-rich foods like chicken, fish, or legumes, they break down into amino acids during digestion, releasing them into the bloodstream at a slow and steady pace. This steady release helps maintain stable blood sugar levels and keeps you feeling full and satisfied, preventing those mid-afternoon energy slumps.

Now, let's talk about teamwork. Imagine your plate as a concert stage. For a harmonious performance, you want a balanced mix of these three macronutrients. Too many carbs without their fat and protein counterparts? That's like a solo act with no backup singers or band. Blood sugar spikes, energy crashes, and hunger strikes. But when you bring them all together, it's a symphony! The carbs provide quick energy, the fats ensure a gradual release, and proteins add the staying power. It's a nutritional masterpiece that keeps your blood sugar levels dancing in perfect rhythm.

In the grand production of your health, understanding the impact of carbohydrates, fats, and proteins on blood sugar is crucial. It's not about banning certain foods or following complicated diets. Instead, it's about creating a culinary masterpiece that nourishes your body, fuels your energy, and keeps the blood sugar concert playing smoothly. So, let's celebrate the diversity on our plates, savor the symphony of flavors, and embrace the magic that happens when our food takes center stage in the incredible dance of our bodies.

Sample Meal Plans and Recipes

Embarking on a journey to balance your blood sugar doesn't mean bidding farewell to delicious meals. In fact, it opens the door to a world of vibrant flavors and nourishing ingredients that will leave your taste buds dancing. Let's explore some sample meal plans and recipes designed to keep your blood sugar levels in harmony.

Breakfast Delights:

1. Quinoa Breakfast Bowl:

Start your day with a protein-packed quinoa bowl. Cook quinoa in almond milk, top it with fresh berries, a sprinkle of chia seeds, and a drizzle of honey. It's a delightful mix of textures and flavors that kickstarts your morning with a nutritional boost.

2. Avocado and Egg Toast:

Elevate your classic toast by adding sliced avocado and a poached egg. The healthy fats in avocado coupled with the protein from the egg create a satisfying breakfast that keeps you fueled until lunch.

Lunchtime Feasts:

3. Grilled Chicken Salad with Citrus Vinaigrette:

For a light and refreshing lunch, toss grilled chicken slices with a vibrant mix of leafy greens, cherry tomatoes, cucumber, and bell peppers. Drizzle a zesty citrus vinaigrette for a burst of flavor without compromising your blood sugar balance.

4. Sweet Potato and Chickpea Buddha Bowl:
Craft a nourishing Buddha bowl with roasted sweet potatoes, chickpeas, quinoa, and a colorful assortment of veggies. Top it off with a tahini dressing for a satisfying, nutrient-rich lunch that satisfies both your taste buds and your body's needs.

Dinner Delicacies:
5. Salmon with Garlic Lemon Butter Sauce:
Indulge in a heart-healthy dinner with grilled or baked salmon. The garlic lemon butter sauce adds a burst of flavor without excess sugars. Pair it with roasted Brussels sprouts and quinoa for a well-balanced meal.

6. Cauliflower Fried Rice:
Give a low-carb twist to a classic favorite. Substitute rice with finely chopped cauliflower and stir-fry it with colorful vegetables, lean protein like shrimp or tofu, and a dash of low-sodium soy sauce. It's a guilt-free, savory delight

that won't send your blood sugar on a rollercoaster.

Snack Attack:

7. Greek Yogurt Parfait:

Create a satisfying snack by layering Greek yogurt with fresh berries, a sprinkle of nuts, and a drizzle of honey. The combination of protein and healthy fats will keep you energized between meals.

8. Veggie Sticks with Hummus:

Snack smart by dipping colorful vegetable sticks into homemade hummus. The fiber in veggies combined with the protein-rich hummus creates a satisfying and blood sugar-friendly snack.

Dessert Dreams:

9. Berry and Chia Seed Pudding:

Satisfy your sweet tooth with a guilt-free berry and chia seed pudding. Mix chia seeds with almond milk and let it set overnight. Top it with a medley of berries for a delightful dessert that won't spike your blood sugar.

10. Dark Chocolate Avocado Mousse:
Indulge in a rich and creamy chocolate mousse made with ripe avocados and dark chocolate. It's a decadent treat that also contributes healthy fats to your diet.

These sample meal plans and recipes aren't just about balancing blood sugar; they're about celebrating the joy of nourishing your body with wholesome, delicious food. So, roll up your sleeves, hit the kitchen, and let your culinary adventure begin!

Chapter 5: Exercise and Blood Sugar Control

How Physical Activity Can Positively Influence Blood Sugar Levels

Alright, buckle up, because we're about to dive into the world of sweat, heartbeats, and blood sugar tango! Picture this: your body is a finely tuned orchestra, and exercise is the conductor waving the baton, keeping everything harmonized, especially that tricky blood sugar rhythm.

Now, let's talk about the superhero of this chapter: physical activity. It's not just about pumping iron in the gym (although that's cool too), but any movement that gets your heart pumping and muscles working. From a brisk walk to a dance-off in your living room, it all counts.

So, why is this physical activity thing such a big deal for your blood sugar? Well, think of it as a magical spell that helps your body use glucose more efficiently. When you get moving, your muscles become sugar sponges, soaking up glucose like a thirsty plant after a rainstorm. But it's not just a one-time deal; regular exercise improves your body's sensitivity to insulin, the blood sugar maestro.

Aerobic exercises, like jogging or swimming, are like the rockstars of blood sugar control. They not only burn calories but also enhance insulin action. It's like giving your insulin a megaphone, helping it shout, "Hey, glucose, get in here and do your thing!" Resistance training, on the other hand, strengthens your muscles, turning them into powerhouse glucose consumers.

But wait, there's more! Exercise isn't just about the immediate effects; it leaves a lasting impact on your blood sugar. Imagine it as a guardian angel, standing watch even when you're resting. Regular physical activity helps maintain stable blood sugar levels throughout the day and improves your body's ability to handle those unexpected sugar spikes.

And here's the best part: you don't need to be an Olympic athlete to reap the rewards. Find something you love, whether it's salsa dancing, hiking, or even chasing after your dog in the backyard. The key is consistency – making movement a part of your daily routine.

So, in a nutshell, when it comes to blood sugar, exercise isn't just a suggestion; it's a celebration of your body's fantastic abilities. It's not about punishment; it's a dance, a joyous movement that keeps your blood sugar grooving to the right beat.

Recommended Exercise For Individuals With Different Fitness Levels

Exercise is like a wardrobe - one size doesn't fit all! Whether you're a gym buff or a couch enthusiast, finding the right exercise groove is like discovering your fashion style. Let's tailor-fit the workout experience for different fitness levels.

For the Newbies:
If the gym feels like a foreign planet, start with the basics. Walking is a game-changer. It's simple, yet it gets the job done. Lace up those sneakers, hit the pavement, and let your journey begin. Add some light bodyweight exercises, like squats and lunges, to spice things up. Think of it as the 'Casual Friday' of workouts – comfortable and not too serious.

The Weekend Warriors:
You've got a day job, but you also rock that yoga mat on the weekends. Variety is the spice of life for you. Mix cardio with strength training to keep things interesting. Try cycling, swimming, or even a dance class to get your heart pumping. Throw in some dumbbells for those biceps, and

voila – you're the James Bond of workouts, suave and versatile.

The Fitness Fanatics:

For those who practically live in their workout gear, it's all about the challenge. High-intensity interval training (HIIT) is your jam. Burpees, sprints, and mountain climbers – you thrive on pushing your limits. Add in some heavy lifting for that extra adrenaline kick. You're the superhero of workouts, conquering every set and rep like a boss.

The Zen Seekers:

If the sound of weights hitting the gym floor is your nightmare, welcome to the zen zone. Yoga and Pilates are your sanctuary. Embrace the tranquility of slow, controlled movements. Stretch, breathe, and find your inner peace. It's like a workout and a spa day rolled into one – the ultimate self-care routine.

The Team Players:

Solo workouts? No thanks. You thrive on the camaraderie of team sports. Join a local soccer league, basketball game, or even a dance crew. You'll not only break a sweat but also make lifelong friends. It's not just exercise; it's a social event – the ultimate win-win.

In the grand symphony of fitness, every instrument plays a vital role. The key is to find your melody – the workout that resonates with your soul.

Benefits of Incorporating Both Aerobic and Resistance Training

Engaging in both aerobic and resistance training offers a dynamic duo of benefits that go beyond just breaking a sweat. Aerobic exercise, like running or dancing, gets your heart pumping and your blood flowing. It's the cardio hero that torches calories, strengthens your cardiovascular system, and boosts overall endurance. But let's not forget the unsung hero: resistance training.

This is the muscle-making powerhouse that involves lifting weights or using your body weight for exercises like squats and push-ups.

Firstly, aerobic exercise is the mood-boosting maestro. Ever notice how a brisk walk or a lively dance session can turn a gloomy day into a sunshine-infused escapade? That's the magic of aerobic workouts releasing endorphins, the brain's natural mood lifters. They're like happiness confetti for your brain. Plus, aerobic exercise enhances lung capacity and heart health, creating a symphony of benefits for your entire cardiovascular system.

Now, let's talk muscles. Resistance training isn't just for the bodybuilder types; it's a secret weapon for everyone. It's like putting your muscles through a strength boot camp. By challenging your muscles with resistance, whether it's lifting dumbbells or using resistance bands, you're sculpting a lean, mean machine. And here's a fun fact – more muscle means a faster metabolism. So, while you're lifting those weights, you're also turning your body into a calorie-burning furnace, even when you're Netflix-and-chilling.

The combination of both aerobic and resistance training creates a tag team effect for weight management. Aerobic workouts help burn calories during the exercise session, while the muscle-building magic of resistance training continues the calorie-torching long after you've hit the shower. It's like having a fitness squad that works around the clock to keep you in shape.

But it's not just about looks and mood – it's about the long game. Aerobic and resistance training together form an unbeatable alliance against chronic conditions. They team up to regulate blood sugar levels, improve insulin sensitivity, and keep your heart in tip-top shape. It's a powerhouse partnership that's not just about fitting into skinny jeans; it's about living your best, healthiest life.

So, when you lace up those running shoes or grab those dumbbells, know that you're not just working out; you're unleashing a double dose of goodness for your body and mind. It's not a battle between cardio and weights; it's a love story – a love story between you and your well-being.

Chapter 6: Lifestyle Changes for Blood Sugar Balance

Importance of Sleep, Hydration, and other Lifestyle Factors.

Getting your blood sugar in check isn't just about counting carbs or hitting the gym. It's a holistic journey, and in this chapter, we're going to explore the unsung heroes: quality sleep, proper hydration, and mastering the art of stress management.

Quality Sleep: The Silent Blood Sugar Regulator

Ever had a night of tossing and turning only to find yourself craving sugary treats the next day? Your body was trying to tell you something. Quality sleep is like a backstage pass to the concert of blood sugar balance. When you're sleep-deprived, your body gets stressed, leading to increased levels of cortisol, the infamous stress hormone. Elevated cortisol can throw your blood sugar out of whack, making those midnight cravings a reality. So, dive into those cozy sheets, embrace the tranquility, and let your body do its nightly dance of restoration.

Proper Hydration: Nectar for Your Blood Sugar Garden

Imagine your blood vessels as a garden, and water as the nourishment it craves. Dehydration is like leaving that garden thirsty, making it harder for your blood sugar to flow smoothly. When you're well-hydrated, your blood becomes a well-tended landscape, supporting efficient insulin function. Hydration isn't just about chugging water; it's about making your blood vessels flourish. So, sip on that water like it's the elixir of life – because, for your blood sugar, it kind of is.

Stress Management: The Zen Master's Guide to Balanced Blood Sugar

Stress — the silent saboteur of blood sugar harmony. When life throws curveballs, your body responds by releasing glucose into the bloodstream, a primitive survival mechanism. In today's world, it's not sabertooth tigers that stress us out, but endless to-do lists and never-ending notifications. Enter stress management: the Zen master's guide to balanced blood sugar. Whether it's a few minutes of deep breathing, a mindful walk, or even a good belly laugh, finding your stress-busting ritual is key to keeping those blood sugar levels in check.

.

The Power of Lifestyle Harmony:

Now, imagine your lifestyle as a symphony. Quality sleep, hydration, and stress management are the conductors orchestrating the sweet melody of balanced blood sugar. When they work together, it's like a harmonious masterpiece – your body humming along in perfect tune.

Think of it this way: skipping sleep, neglecting water, and letting stress run rampant is like throwing a wild party in your body. The result? Blood sugar chaos, mood swings, and a body that's on the brink of a rebellion.

But when you prioritize sleep like a precious gem, keep the water flowing like a serene river, and show stress the exit door, you're creating an environment where your blood sugar can dance to its natural rhythm.

So, here's your mission: turn your bedroom into a sleep sanctuary, keep that water bottle by your side like a loyal companion, and show stress the exit like a bouncer at the hottest club in town. Your blood sugar will be doing the happy dance in no time.

Remember, it's not about drastic changes but weaving these habits into the fabric of your daily life. Let's make lifestyle changes that feel less like a chore and more like a celebration of your body's incredible dance with balance. Cheers to sweet dreams, hydrated days, and a stress-free dance floor for your blood sugar!

Practical Tips for Incorporating Healthy Habits Into Daily Life

Transforming your daily routine to support blood sugar balance doesn't have to be a monumental task—it's all about weaving practical habits seamlessly into your life. Here are some down-to-earth tips to make these lifestyle changes a seamless part of your day:

1. Morning Mindfulness Rituals:
Start your day with a few moments of mindfulness. Before the hustle begins, sit quietly, focus on your breath, or express gratitude. It sets a positive tone, calming your nervous system and gearing you up for the day ahead.

2. Hydration Hacks:

Turn hydration into a delightful routine. Keep a reusable water bottle by your side, infusing it with slices of citrus, cucumber, or a sprig of mint. This not only makes water more appealing but also adds a hint of flavor without any added sugars.

3. Office Ergonomics and Micro-Movement:

If you're tied to a desk, make it work for you. Adjust your chair and monitor to ergonomic perfection. Set a timer for every hour as a cue to stretch or take a brisk walk. Micro-movements keep your metabolism active, preventing blood sugar spikes.

4. Snack Smartly:

Snacking is an art. Keep a stash of nuts, seeds, or veggies at arm's reach. When hunger strikes, you're armed with wholesome options. It curbs the temptation to reach for less blood-sugar-friendly treats.

5. Lunchtime Power Walks:

Use your lunch break for more than just eating. Take a brisk walk outside. The fresh air and movement contribute to better digestion and help stabilize blood sugar levels. Plus, it's a natural mood booster.

6. Stress-Busting Breathing Breaks:

Incorporate mini-breathing breaks into your routine. When stress creeps in, pause. Take slow, deep breaths. It instantly calms the nervous system, reducing the release of stress hormones that can impact blood sugar.

7. Evening Unplugging Ritual:

Make a tech-free zone at least an hour before going to bed. The blue light emitted by screens can disrupt sleep patterns, affecting blood sugar regulation. Opt for a calming activity like reading or gentle stretching to ease into a restful night.

8. Sleep Sanctuary:

Make your bedroom a sanctuary for quality sleep. Invest in comfortable bedding, keep the room cool and dark, and establish a consistent sleep schedule. Quality sleep is a cornerstone of balanced blood sugar.

9. Gratitude Journaling:

Finish the day by writing down a few things you're thankful for. This simple practice shifts your focus to the positive, reducing overall stress levels and promoting better blood sugar control.

These small tweaks to your daily routine can create a ripple effect, positively influencing your blood sugar balance without disrupting your life. Remember, it's the everyday habits that add up to a revolutionary change.

Chapter 7: Mindful Living and Stress Reduction

In this Chapter, we're diving into the fascinating realm of Mindful Living and Stress Reduction, where we unravel the intricate dance between stress and blood sugar levels. Picture this: your body is like a finely tuned orchestra, with blood sugar playing a pivotal role in the symphony of your well-being.

The Connection Between Stress and Blood Sugar Levels

Stress, that sneaky little troublemaker, has more influence on your blood sugar than you might think. When stress barges in uninvited, it sets off a domino effect within your body. First, the adrenal glands release adrenaline, gearing you up for a fight-or-flight situation. Now, here's the twist – adrenaline triggers the release of glucose into your bloodstream. It's like your body thinks you're about to run from a bear, even if you're just stressed about a looming deadline.

But that's not the end of the story. Cortisol, another stress hormone, enters the scene. While adrenaline is the sprinter, cortisol is the marathon runner. It hangs around longer, encouraging your body to replenish the energy it just burned. How does it do that? By craving sugary, high-energy foods. Suddenly, that chocolate bar or bag of chips becomes irresistible – blame it on cortisol.

Now, imagine this happening repeatedly, day in and day out. Chronic stress becomes a relentless conductor, orchestrating a continuous surge of glucose into your bloodstream. The result? Elevated blood sugar levels, paving the way for potential health issues down the road.

But fear not – the Glucose Revolution offers a backstage pass to disrupting this stress-induced symphony. Mindful living takes center stage. Picture yourself in a serene meadow, not a care in the world. Mindfulness techniques, like deep breathing and meditation, become your anti-stress maestros. They signal to your body that it's okay to put the brakes on the glucose release, calming the storm of stress hormones.

By weaving mindfulness into your daily tapestry, you're not just managing stress; you're redefining your body's response to it. It's like giving your orchestra a new set of instruments, transforming chaotic discord into a harmonious melody. As stress loses its grip, so does its impact on your blood sugar levels.

So, here's the deal: embrace the art of mindful living. Turn down the volume on stress, and watch as your blood sugar levels follow suit. It's a dance between serenity and physiology, and you're the lead choreographer in this extraordinary performance.

Mindfulness Techniques and Stress Reduction Strategies

In our fast-paced lives, stress can sometimes feel like an unwelcome companion. But fear not – the world of mindfulness and stress reduction offers a treasure trove of techniques to help you find calm amidst the chaos

1. Breathe In, Breathe Out: It sounds basic, right? But consciously focusing on your breath can be a game-changer. Take a slow, deep breath in through your nose, hold it for a moment, and then exhale gently through your mouth. Feel the rhythm and repeat. It's a simple act that can bring you back to the present moment, away from the chaotic whirlwind of stress.

2. The Art of Observation: Mindfulness is about paying attention, and not just to your thoughts. Observe your surroundings, and notice the subtle details you often overlook. Feel the warmth of the sun on your skin, listen to the rustle of leaves, or appreciate the colors around you. Engaging your senses in the present moment is a quick ticket to stress reduction.

3. Mindful Walking: Take a stroll, not to get somewhere, but to be somewhere. Pay attention to the sensation of your feet meeting the ground, the movement of your body, and the rhythm of your steps. Let your mind wander without fixating on any particular thought. It's a walking meditation, and it's surprisingly effective.

4. Unplug and Reconnect: In a world buzzing with notifications, sometimes the best stress reduction technique is to unplug. Put away the screens, even if it's just for a short while. Instead, engage in a real, uninterrupted conversation, or spend quality time with a hobby. The digital detox can work wonders.

5. Gratitude Journaling: Shift your focus from what's stressing you to what you're grateful for. Begin a thankfulness diary and write down three things you're grateful for every day. It can be as simple as a hot cup of coffee in the morning or a smile from a stranger. Shifting your mindset from stress to gratitude rewires your brain for positivity.

6. Progressive Muscle Relaxation: Stress often manifests physically. Progressive muscle relaxation involves tensing and then slowly releasing each muscle group, starting from your toes and working your way up. It not only eases physical tension but also calms the mind.

7. Mindful Eating: Turn your mealtime into a mindful experience. Engage your senses as you savor each bite. Notice the flavors, textures, and smells. This not only makes eating more enjoyable but also helps you avoid stress-induced binge eating.

In the hustle of life, these simple, everyday mindfulness techniques act as anchors, grounding you in the present. Incorporate them into your routine, and let the stress melt away like ice cream on a sunny day.

Importance of Mental Well-Being in Overall Health.

Mental well-being is like the hidden architect behind the scenes of our overall health, silently pulling the strings and orchestrating the grand symphony of our lives. It's not just about keeping a serene facade; it's the secret sauce that flavors every aspect of our existence.

Picture this: your mind is the control center, the epicenter of your daily operations. When it's running smoothly, everything else falls into place. Just as a gardener tends to the soil before planting seeds, nurturing mental well-being is the foundation upon which the garden of our overall health blossoms.

Our minds are remarkable multitaskers. They navigate the ebbs and flows of life, weathering storms and basking in sunshine. Mental well-being isn't just about the absence of stress or the occasional blues; it's about cultivating resilience in the face of life's inevitable challenges. It's like having a sturdy umbrella in a sudden downpour - you might still get wet, but you won't be swept away by the tempest.

Let's not forget the interconnected dance between mental and physical health. It's not a solo performance; it's a duet where each partner influences the other. Stress, anxiety, and negative thoughts can cast a shadow over physical well-being, affecting everything from sleep patterns to immune function. On the flip side, a buoyant mental state can infuse energy into your physical being, giving you the zest to tackle the day.

Think of mental well-being as the captain steering the ship of your overall health through the unpredictable seas of life. It's not about being perpetually happy; it's about having a compass that helps you navigate the highs and lows with grace. When your mental well-being is in sync, you're better equipped to adapt to life's twists and turns.

In this fast-paced world, where we're often juggling a multitude of responsibilities, neglecting mental well-being is akin to driving a car without ever checking the engine. It might work for a while, but sooner or later, the wear and tear catches up. Prioritizing mental health isn't a luxury; it's a fundamental investment in our longevity and vitality.

So, here's to tending to the garden within, nurturing the captain at the helm, and embracing the profound truth that mental well-being isn't just a piece of the health puzzle; it's the masterpiece that completes the picture.

Conclusion

As we wrap up our journey through the Glucose Revolution, it's crucial to remember that balancing blood sugar is more than a destination; it's a continuous, dynamic journey. Think of it as a road trip where the landscape changes, and you adapt to the twists and turns. The key lies in taking small, manageable steps rather than trying to sprint towards a finish line that doesn't exist.

Picture this journey as a series of scenic rest stops. Each chapter in this book has been one of those stops, offering you insights, tools, and a roadmap for maintaining balanced blood sugar. But here's the secret: the real magic happens between those stops, in the everyday choices and actions you make. It's in the morning ritual of choosing a nutrient-packed breakfast, the decision to take a brisk walk during lunch, and the conscious effort to unwind and destress in the evening.

Balancing blood sugar isn't about perfection; it's about progress. It's about finding joy in the process, discovering what works for you, and celebrating the victories—no matter how small. Remember, Rome wasn't built in a day, and your health journey won't be either. You're building a foundation for a healthier, more vibrant life, one choice at a time.

As you embark on this journey, let hope be your constant companion. Hope is the fuel that propels you forward, even when the road gets a bit bumpy. Believe in the transformative power of the choices you make today, and trust that those choices will create a ripple effect of positive change.

Empowerment is the heartbeat of this journey. It's the realization that you have the ability to influence your health destiny. You're not a passive traveler; you're the driver of your own wellness adventure. Embrace this power, relish in the autonomy of your decisions, and savor the delicious moments of self-discovery along the way.

So, here's to you—the intrepid explorer of your health and well-being. May your journey be filled with joy, resilience, and a deep sense of accomplishment. As you take those small steps, know that you're not just balancing blood sugar; you're crafting a narrative of vitality, a story that unfolds uniquely and beautifully with each chapter of your life. Cheers to your journey, and may it be as extraordinary as you are!

9 798876 351111